HEALTHY LIVING

Change Your Lifestyle, Change Your Life

KATHERINE YOUNG

Legal & Disclaimer

The information contained in this book and its contents is not designed to replace or take the place of any form of medical or professional advice and is not meant to replace the need for independent medical, financial, legal or other professional advice or services, as may be required. The content and information in this book have been provided for educational and entertainment purposes only.

The content and information contained in this book have been compiled from sources deemed reliable, and it is accurate to the best of the Author's knowledge, information, and belief. However, the Author cannot guarantee its accuracy and validity and cannot be held liable for any errors and/or omissions. Further, changes are periodically made to this book as and when needed. Where appropriate and/or necessary, you must consult a professional (including but not limited to your doctor, attorney, financial advisor or such other professional advisor) before using any of the suggested remedies, techniques, or information in this book.

Upon using the contents and information contained in this book, you agree to hold harmless the Author from and against any damages, costs, and expenses, including any legal fees potentially resulting from the application of any of the information provided by this book. This disclaimer applies to any loss, damages or injury caused by the use and application, whether directly or indirectly, of any advice or information presented, whether for breach of contract, tort, negligence, personal injury, criminal intent, or under any other cause of action.
You agree to accept all risks of using the information presented inside this book.

You agree that by continuing to read this book, where appropriate and/or necessary, you shall consult a professional (including but not limited to your doctor, attorney, or financial advisor or such other advisor as needed) before using any of the suggested remedies, techniques, or information in this book.

Table of Contents

Healthy Living

Introduction

We should constantly improve and take action to have a healthy lifestyle. To most people, healthy living means that both physical and mental health is in balance for a person. Being in good health does not only prevent us from diseases, but it also improves our mental and physical health. There are also many diets that can help us live a healthy life. There are many ways to be healthy including eating healthy, physical activities, stress management, and weight management.

We should avoid unhealthy foods (and junk food) which are harmful to our health. This includes food and drinks high in sugar, low in nutrients and high in calories. Eating these foods on a regular basis can lead to health problems such as cardiovascular disease, diabetes and increased risk of obesity. Additionally, we should also refrain from tobacco and alcohol.

1. Physical activity:

We can maintain and improve our health through physical activity. According to researchers, adults ages 16-84 should do at least 150 minutes of moderate activity or 75 minutes of vigorous activity. That activity may be an aerobic physical activity, simple exercise or a walk. This physical activity can improve cardiorespiratory and muscular fitness as well as improve bone health and reduce the risk of depression.

2. Healthy diet:

A healthy diet is vital for healthy living, so we should avoid junk food and eat more vegetables and fruits and fewer carbohydrates and foods that are high in sodium. We should also incorporate lean meat, poultry, beans, eggs, and nuts into a healthy diet. We should avoid trans carbohydrates and fatty foods.

We are aware that tobacco use has negative effects on human health, not only to the smoker but to non-smokers due to secondhand smoke. Tobacco use leads to diseases affecting the heart, liver, and lungs. Thus, to have a healthy life, you should avoid smoking. When you live a healthy life, you will not be susceptible to diseases. Healthy living is essential for a long life.

Chapter 1
How to Change Your Habits

What is habit – good habit or bad habit? Habits are, "routines of behavior that are repeated regularly and tend to occur subconsciously," according to Wikipedia; while according to Macmillan Dictionary, habit is, "something that you do often or regularly, often without thinking about it." Good habits are beneficial to us as they will help us to be disciplined and have self-control. Habits like exercise, consumption of alcohol in moderation, and a balanced diet lead us to a healthy lifestyle.

A bad habit is a negative behavior pattern, e.g., nail-biting, spending too much time watching television or using a computer, using tobacco or smoking excessively. We should find ways to change our habits by identifying the habit we want to change and then consciously choose different behavior. We should replace the unhealthy/bad habits with healthy habits. This will benefit us in the long run.

It is not easy to identify bad habits that have been part of your daily routine for many years. Bad habits usually have many triggers. For example, when I want to quit drinking, I will take note of all triggers to urge me to drink like stress, eating, frustrations, and type of company. Anytime a trigger(s) happens, replace it with a new habit. Remember, it can take some time to change your habits so be patient and kind to yourself.

## 1.	Some Unhealthy Habits:

There are many unhealthy habits we have adopted that have made our bodies unhealthy and lead to increased risk of diseases such as obesity, and chronic diseases like type 2 diabetes and cardiovascular disease.

Some of these unhealthy habits are:

- Lack of exercise

- Poor food choices

- Alcohol consumption

- Bad sleeping habits

- Eating junk food

If the above habits form part of your routine, you may need to gently, slowly change to a healthier lifestyle. Replace the above unhealthy habits with good habits, and after you have done that many times, eventually the new good habit will be automatic and become part of your daily routine.

2. Little Habits That Can Change Your Life:

Sometimes, it is tough for us to maintain a good habit, but if you put your mind to it anything is possible. You can adopt positive habits to make changes that will positively impact your life.

i. Focus on One Goal:

You may have many goals that you want to achieve, but to succeed in all of them you will need to focus on one goal at a time and see it through until you achieve it. This way, you are giving your energy and time to one purpose only. For example, if you have three goals in your life, then you must pick one goal and focus on it. When one goal is completed, only then can you move to the next goal. For example, if you want to lose weight, you will need to change your eating habits, eat in moderation and exercise regularly until you have lost the amount of weight that you want, e.g., 10kg. Then you move on to lose more weight, say another 20kg. When you have the will power, you will surely find ways to reshape your lifestyle habits to help you achieve lasting change, and ultimately, your goal.

ii. Kindness:

Kindness is a good habit to inculcate in your heart and in your everyday life. As we all know that when you are kind to everyone, whether it's an animal or a bird or any human being, it also lifts your mood and improves your well-being. Try to be kind and friendly towards everyone. It is a great first step towards changing your lifestyle.

iii. Have a Daily Routine:

When you have a daily routine, it will bring many positive changes in your life. You will feel better and stay confident after making positive changes in your life. It also helps with your mental wellbeing and creativity. Start your day with positive thoughts, set a time to exercise daily and have at least seven to eight hours of sleep every night.

iv.   You Can Change Your Habits:

Changing your habits overnight is difficult. You can always take one step at a time. For example, if you have decided to walk for 100 minutes and you are not able to complete the walk, start with walking for 15 minutes daily and slowly increase by 10 minutes every couple of days until you reach your goal of 100 minutes per day. Take small steps daily and you can achieve your goals as time goes by.

v.   Develop Positive Thinking:

Many books have been published on positive thinking and the effects of developing a positive way of thinking. It is one of the best habits to adopt because it will change your life. When you think positively, it will not only lead you to success but also attract good things in your life. For example, some people drink alcohol in moderate amounts for health benefits, while some drink too much until they are intoxicated or make drinking a bad habit. When you decide to think positively and surround yourself with encouraging family members and friends, you can have the power and determination to quit drinking, but it does take time and practice as you are creating a healthier habit. Always make it a point to look at the positive or brighter side of life; this will enable you to cope better with stressful situations, live healthier lifestyles, get more physical activity and follow a healthier diet.

vi.   Exercise:

Everyone knows the importance of exercise and that it has many benefits for your body and helps to combat diseases. Everyone should maintain a regular exercise routine and keep as active as possible. There are many types of exercise that you can take up. You do not need to do intense workouts. You can start off with easy exercises like swimming, walking or easy stretching exercises. You can feel many positive changes in your body when you make it a habit of doing exercise daily, such as a decrease in stress levels, and it is also beneficial for mental health. Exercise can improve your health and help reduce the risk of many diseases like diabetes and cardiovascular diseases.

Chapter 2

How to Change Your Life Through Healthy Living

When you make changes to daily aspects of your life, such as how to spend time, to schedule your day or when to eat. These are all lifestyle changes that can make you healthy and positively affect your life. It all depends on your choices and priorities. Your priorities always decide how fit you are and how successful you are.

1.   Stay Organized:

You must stay organized for a healthy lifestyle change to occur. Organized means having a tidy desk, prepared meals, painted nails, planned things. As we all know, if you remain neat and orderly it has a significant impact on your personality. It only takes 10 to 15 minutes a day to stay organized.

2.   Wake Up Early in the Morning:

My grandmother always advises me to wake up early in the morning as it is an excellent habit. Waking up early sets the tone for the day, makes you feel organized and productive and improves concentration. Early risers tend to eat breakfast while late risers tend to skip breakfast, which will lead to poorer eating habits later in the day.

The good thing about waking up early is that you get enough time for all the tasks you must perform during the day. It is sad to say that in this modern world, most people wake up late in the morning around 11 am or 12 noon.

This is because of the media and the internet. I am not against it, but you must spend your time wisely on the internet. Going to sleep early and waking up early will help you make use of the positive change in your life.

3.   Morning routine:

A morning routine is essential for your everyday life. When you develop the habit of waking up early, then it will be easier for you to have a morning routine to motivate you for the whole day. You have time for self-development and fitness. You should make time for some simple exercises, such as walking for at least 15 minutes, as morning exercises will keep you energized all day long. You can also set aside some time to enjoy the peace and quiet of the morning and find that your daily commute is easier with less traffic on the road.

4. Show Your Creativity:

Creativity is a great habit to develop for yourself. Some people like to write, and some people like to paint. Both are creative things that you can also do. Doing creative things will inculcate a positive attitude in your personality, and you will be more confident than before. You can also show your creativity through coloring books, painting nails, playing with makeup, taking photos, filming, drawing, editing and much more. Creativity reduces stress and keeps you healthy. Creativity is important as it boosts self-confidence, stimulates the brain and is fun and enjoyable. We all need time to rest, rejuvenate and do something fun and stimulating. So, block off some time each day or week for a little creativity.

5.   Eating Healthy Stuff:

Eating healthy is important as good nutrition is an important part of a healthy lifestyle. Together with physical activity, it can help you maintain a healthy weight, reduce your risk of chronic diseases and promote your overall health. We see junk food everywhere – in fast food restaurants, grocery and convenience stores. This refers to foods that contribute lots of calories but little nutritional value. Junk foods tend to lead to overeating, and they tend to replace other more nutritious food. We should eat healthy food like fruits, vegetables, and nuts. You do not need to eliminate foods you enjoy as this usually leads to cheating or giving up on your new eating plan. Make a few small changes at a time. Your small changes can become your habits, then you can continue to add more healthy choices.

My suggestion is that you should prepare more of your own meals. In this way, you can take charge of what you are eating and are able to monitor exactly what goes into your food. Remember to drink plenty of water as it helps to flush our systems of waste products and toxins.

6.   Slow Down and Reflect on the Moment:

In this busy world, we focus too much on our jobs, work and everyday tasks that we forget the beautiful moments in life which we should be experiencing.

Life is short. It passes by very quickly. You should slow down and enjoy life without sacrificing your goals and plans. So, start right now … ask yourself "What is life to you?" Is it about doing less? Or being able to spend more quality time with your family or loved ones or even friends? Make time through time management and planning as slowing down is a conscious choice, you need to be mindful of whatever you are doing at the moment. Focus on what is going on right now.

It will be great for you and your loved ones to pass the day by going to a calm and relaxed place. You should appreciate the beauty of the world, the happiness of the children, the love of your soulmate, or a great chat with your friends. You should analyze things and beauty more innovatively. In other words, you should enjoy every moment of life.

7.   Long Term Health:

A healthy lifestyle has both short- and long-term health benefits. You can achieve this when you eat healthy food, get plenty of sleep, exercise, and drink a lot of water. These are some of the things that can add years to your life and reduce the risk of certain diseases including cancer, diabetes, cardiovascular disease, and obesity. You should slowly eliminate smoking or drinking alcohol. In the short-term, it can make you feel better and give you more energy.

You should maintain a healthy weight, and if you are overweight, you can successfully lose weight through exercising at least 30 minutes a day as part of a daily routine.

Remember to drink plenty of water as adult humans are 60 percent water and our blood is 90 percent water. It is commonly recommended to drink eight 8-ounce glasses of water per day (the 8x8 rule). Water is involved in many important functions, including:

- flushing out waste from your body
- regulating body temperature
- helping your brain function

8.   Read Your Beauty Labels:

In the US, researchers have found 1 of every 8 ingredients used in cosmetics is an industrial chemical. Due to very loose regulations, products can still be full of toxic chemicals and other harmful ingredients. The only way to avoid being duped is to read the labels and to make sure you really understand what you are putting on your face and are making the healthiest decision for your body and the environment.

You need to stay away from beauty products that have chemicals; look for the natural and organic brands which have simple ingredients like coconut oil or lavender. Be aware that there may be unscrupulous manufacturers who will mislead their customers with false labels.

Chapter 3
Fitness and Exercise

Fitness and exercise are very important ways to make positive changes in your life. In this stressful life, exercise has proven to release stress and help the body invigorate. The first thing about fitness and exercise is that you must make the decision to want to be healthy You should persevere to achieve your goal. If you are moving towards fitness and exercise, ultimately you are improving your health and reduce your risk of all kinds of diseases.

1.   How Exercise Affects Your Fitness:

During exercise, our muscles require more blood flow and oxygen. Your muscles become stronger. It also trains your heart to work more efficiently. Your lung health will also increase with the help of fitness. During exercise, our brain also releases chemicals called endorphins which alter the mood of the person.

Our bones also become healthy from exercise. In other words, we can say that all muscles become stronger with exercise. You are using your muscles when you are in a continuous activity like walking, jogging, cycling, or dancing.

2.   Best Exercises to Keep You Fit:

i.   Walking:

As we all know that walking is the primary exercise; also called cardiovascular exercise. The good thing about walking is that it burns calories in a very organized manner and strengthens the heart. You can walk anywhere, anytime. You just need a pair of shoes and then you can start walking. Physicians recommend a minimum of 30 minutes of exercise on most days of the week.

ii.   Push-Ups:

Push-ups are also a very useful exercise as they strengthen the chest, triceps, shoulders, and even the core trunk muscles all at once. The good thing about pushups is that you can try them at any level of fitness. Start by kneeling on an exercise mat or floor. Place your hands slightly wider than shoulder-width apart with fingers facing forward. You should make a perfect diagonal with your body. Now, lift your body by bending and straightening your elbows. Then move down and up and make a perfect rhythm of push-ups. An alternative position is to bend your legs at the knees so you do not have to lift your whole body.

iii.   Rotation:

Rotation is a simple exercise that everyone can do anywhere and anytime. All you do is stand tall with good alignment. Then you should hold a weight or a magnetic ball. Then stretch your arms in front of you holding the weight.

Moving side to side, rotate the ball as much as your mobility allows. Make sure that you are maintaining a good posture. Rotation is a very good exercise as it will work on your waist and lower body. When you carry on this exercise regularly, then ultimately you will lose fat from your waist and lower body.

iv.   Lunges:

Lunges help improve your balance. They also increase the strength of your legs and can promote functional movement in your body. You can do this exercise by standing with your feet shoulder-width apart and arms down on your sides. Now, take a step forward with your right leg and the left leg in a backward position. Now, repeat the same process with your left leg.

v.   Sit-Ups:

This exercise is a basic exercise and it is very effective at targeting the abdominal muscles. The person who has lower back problems can start these sit-ups and stick with it since it requires just your upper back and shoulders to lift off the floor. Lie on the floor with your knees in an upward position and have your hands behind your head. The crunch requires your upper back and shoulders to lift off the ground. Do not strain your neck when you lift your upper body from the floor.

3.   Benefits of exercise:

Regular exercise of 30 minutes of moderate-intensity physical activity on most days, if not daily, and physical activity may help you in many ways:

- Help you control your weight
- Reduce your risk of heart disease
- Help your body manage blood sugar and insulin levels
- Help you quit smoking
- Improve your mental health and mood
- Improve your sleep
- Increase your chances of living longer

Ultimately, you are the most important person in your life. Take care of yourself. Once your health goes, there goes your ability to take care of your loved ones and others.

4.   Controlling the Weight:

You can control weight with the help of exercise and lose weight by burning your calories. If you are not able to exercise every day, do not worry as any activity is better than none. You can climb the stairs instead of the elevator or go for longer walks. Exercise helps with maintaining a healthy weight as well as maintaining mobility in your spine.

5.   Stay Away from Diseases:

You can stay away from many diseases with the help of exercise. When you do exercise and physical activities regularly, you can reduce the risk of health problems like type 2 diabetes, depression, anxiety, cancer, arthritis, metabolic syndrome, stroke, and high blood pressure.

6.   Exercise Improves Mood:

Exercises or any kind of physical activity, besides making you energized, will stimulate different types of brain chemicals. Hormones like endorphins released during exercise will make you feel happier, more relaxed, and less anxious. Therefore, you are in a good mood after exercise. Exercises make a good form of therapy for people suffering from anxiety or depression

7.   Exercise Promotes Better Sleep:

There are many people who are not able to sleep well at night. Regular exercise helps you sleep better by making you feel tired before you sleep. Exercise helps you fall asleep faster and even helps you stay asleep during the night. Researchers have also found that exercise can increase a person's total sleep time when done consistently. Be mindful not to exercise too close to bedtime as you may be too energized to fall asleep. Body temperature stays elevated for about four hours after you finish exercising. Higher body temperature can interfere with your ability to sleep. Regular exercise also helps to regulate your body's circadian rhythm (internal clock).

8.   Exercise Boosts Energy

With the help of regular exercise, your body delivers more oxygen and nutrients to your tissues, and your cardiovascular system also works very efficiently. This can improve your muscle strength and boost your endurance. Now you have more energy to handle daily chores. Your heart and lungs also become healthy with the help of exercise.

Chapter 4
Food and Diet Tips

There are many food and diet tips that will help you remain healthy and lively. All you must do is to eat the right number of calories. With the help of healthy eating, you can maintain the balance between the energy you consume and the energy you use. You will gain more weight when you drink or eat more than your body needs because it remains in the body as stored fat.

1.   Eat Lots of Fruits and Vegetables:

It is recommended to eat five portions of a variety of fruit and vegetables every day. You can eat the fruits and vegetables in canned, dried, juiced, frozen, or fresh forms. You should eat 80 grams of fresh, canned, or frozen fruits and vegetables and 30 grams of a portion of the dry fruit.

2.   Eat More Fish:

As we all know, fish is a very good source of protein. It also contains many vitamins and minerals. You should eat fish twice a week and at least 1 portion of oily fish. Oily fish has Omega 3 fats in it, which may prevent heart disease.

3.   Eat High Fiber Starchy Carbohydrates:

You usually eat potatoes, bread, pasta, rice, and cereals. They all are starchy carbohydrates. You should choose high fiber or whole grain carbohydrates like brown rice, potatoes with their skin, and whole wheat pasta. Make sure that you do not stick to the refined starchy carbohydrates. In fact, try the whole grain varieties. Avoid carbohydrates that have fats like oils on chips, butter on bread, or pasta which is rich in creamy sauces.

4.   Avoid Using Saturated Fat and Sugar:

Fats are also important for your diet, but keep in mind the types and amount of fats. As many of us know, there are two types of fats: Saturated and Unsaturated. Saturated fats are not healthy as they increase the amount of cholesterol in the body and the risk of developing heart diseases. So, we should go for unsaturated fats like a small amount of vegetable oil, olive oil, or reduced-fat, ghee or lean meat. You should cut off any visible fat from the meat. You should not go for butter, hard cheese, cakes, biscuits, creams, sausages, or fatty cuts of meat because these have saturated fats and are not good for health.

5.   Drink Plenty of Water and Fluids:

You probably have heard the advice, "Drink eight 8-ounce glasses of water a day." That's easy to remember, and it's a reasonable goal to hydrate your body. You may need to adjust the amount of water intake if you exercise, you are in a hot or humid environment, pregnant or breast-feeding. You should avoid sugary, soft and fizzy drinks as it will increase your weight and replace it with water. If you find that water is bland, just add slices of lemon for that extra taste.

6.   Weight Loss Tips to Make Things Better:

i.   Drink Water a Half-Hour Before Meals:

Doctors recommend drinking water a half-hour before meals as it increases the weight loss processes.

ii.   Eat Soluble Fiber:

Fibers are the best way to reduce fat, especially from the abdomen. There are many fiber supplements available to help you lose weight.

iii.   Get a Good Night's Sleep:

You should sleep well in the night as poor sleep increases your risk for weight gain.

iv.   Eat Your Food Slowly:

When you eat your food slowly then it will boost the weight-reducing hormones in your body. You will gain weight at a higher rate if you are a fast eater.

iv.   Eat a High-Protein Breakfast:

Start your day with a high-protein breakfast as it will reduce your cravings and calorie intake throughout the day.

v.   Eat Whole Foods:

You will become healthier when you are eating whole foods as they don't come with an ingredients list. So, you are just nourishing your body with nutrient-dense foods which are also natural.

vi.   Snack Smartly:

Snacks are one of the reasons of people are putting on more weight. You should go for healthy snacks available such as nuts and cut up veggies that can help you stay on track when the craving strikes.

vii.   Types of Food that Will be Helpful in Burning Belly Fat:

There are several delicious foods that can burn your belly fat.

These include:

- Green tea
- Citrus fruits have Vitamin C, which is also in colorful produce like red peppers, and oranges.
- Berries
- Chocolate skim milk
- Yogurt
- Avocados
- Bananas
- Whole Grains

a.   Roasted or grilled food

Many people know that roasted or grilled meat, vegetables, potatoes, seafood are low in calories as it brings out the natural sweetness and flavor in foods. These are rich flavor foods with fewer calories.

b.   Plant Protein Foods:

Beans and peas are plant protein foods. You can also go for soya products and unsalted nuts and seeds.

c.   Dairy Products:

Dairy products, such as cheese, yogurt and low-fat milk, are very important for your body as they will build and maintain strong bones that are needed for everyday activities.

Chapter 5
Fruit Nutrition

Nature has gifted us with lots of fruits, and no one can deny the importance of fruits. Fruits are essential for our health. They are rich in minerals, antioxidants, vitamins, and plant-derived micronutrients. You can see the beauty of fruits as they have beautiful colors. Nuts are also rich in flavors.

They are also high in nutrient profile, and you can become rejuvenated and fit when you eat fruits. They also prevent you from many diseases.

1.   Benefits of Fruits:

i.   Rich in Nutrients and Antioxidants:

Many antioxidants are also present in grains such as polyphenolic flavonoids, Vitamin C, and anthocyanins. With the help of these antioxidants, our body can fight many diseases like cancer.

ii.   Improves the Immune System:

It also improves our immune system and assists the body in developing the capacity to fight against many ailments. The fantastic thing about fruits is that they are low in calories and fat. Fruits are rich in fiber, simple sugars, and vitamins which are very useful for health.

iii.   Removing Cholesterol and Fats from the Body:

There are plenty of soluble dietary fibers present in fruits which place a vital role in removing cholesterol and fats from the body. Therefore, fruits are very helpful in increasing the digestion process. It also prevents people from having constipation problems.

iv.   Blue Fruits:

You can see many blue fruits like blue-black grapes, acai berry, chokeberry, mulberries. The fruits which are a blue or deep purple color have anthocyanins present in them. Anthocyanins contain a polyphenolic compound which is only present in blue fruits. Anthocyanin is a potent antioxidant that is very helpful in removing free radicals from the body. Anthocyanins protect you against many cancers, infections, and aging. These pigments are present just underneath the skin of the fruit.

v.   Protect You from Damage:

Fruits are also rich in vitamins, minerals, micronutrients, and pigment of antioxidants. Thus, fruits are very healthy for the body. These vitamins and nutrients help the body to prevent the natural changes of aging by protecting from damage and rejuvenating cells, tissues, and organs.

2.   Benefits of Dry Fruits:

In dry fruits, there are many vitamins and minerals present. Doctors recommend having dry fruits daily as it enhances the overall bioavailability of nutrients. You can eat dried grapes, raisins, goji berry, apricots, tamarind, and dates. These are rich in calcium, zinc, selenium, iron, and manganese.

You can also mix some dry fruits with fresh fruits because, in fresh fruits, Vitamin C is present, which enhances the absorption of iron inside the stomach. There are some dry fruits that are better than others. First in the list is almonds, then cashews and then walnuts. Then comes raisins, pistachios, and dates. These dry fruits are rich in vitamins and proteins; they also boost immunity and prevent lifestyle diseases such as high cholesterol and diabetes. The best way to include dry fruits in one's daily diet is to use them as snacks or to include them in daily cooking and in various dishes.

3.   Mango:

As we all know, mango is called the king of fruits. It is prevalent all over the world with its unique flavor, fragrance, taste, and health-promoting qualities. There are also many types of mango. An antioxidant, polyphenolic flavonoid is also present in mango along with different vitamins, minerals, and prebiotic dietary fiber. Mangoes are an excellent source of vitamin C.

According to new research, it has been found that mango may protect people from degenerative diseases, including type 2 diabetes and cancer.

4.   Apple:

Apple is the most popular fruit, and this is the favorite fruit of health-conscious people and fitness lovers. Everyone knows about the saying that "an apple a day keeps the doctor away". It is a beautiful fruit with phytonutrients that are optimal for health and wellness.

You can find apples in different colors depending on the cultivator type. There are many antioxidants present in the apple which are responsible for the overall growth and development of the person.

Apples are also rich in dietary fiber. There are no fats and cholesterol in apples, and they are also rich in antioxidant phytonutrients, flavonoids, and polyphenolics. They are also a rich source of tartaric acid which gives the tart flavor to them, and it also prevents the body from harmful effects of free radicals. Apples also have high levels of quercetin, a flavonoid that may have anti-cancer properties.

5.   Banana:

Banana is available in all seasons of the year. Bananas are a rich source of energy and have a fresh and creamy taste. Bananas have easily digestible flesh which is made from simple sugars like glucose and sucrose.

You get instant energy when you eat a single banana. Doctors recommend bananas to the undernourished children so that they can grow. Bananas can have benefits for exercise, blood sugar control, and digestive health. There are polyphenolic antioxidants present in bananas such as lutein, zeaxanthin, alpha, and beta carotene.

Bananas are well known for their high potassium content. A medium banana contains 422 mg, out of the adequate adult intake of 4,500 mg, of potassium. Potassium helps the body control heart rate and blood pressure and helps with regular bowel movements and stomach issues, such as ulcers and colitis.

6.   Grapes:

Grapes are also famous all over the world and have been called the queen of fruits since ancient times. It is also called table fruit. Grapes have many health-promoting polynucleotides such as polyphenolic antioxidants, minerals, and vitamins.

They are many varieties of grapes, such as Thompson seedless, red globe, flame seedless and many more. The polyphenolic phytochemical compound present in grapes called resveratrol. It is a powerful antioxidant and plays a protective role against colon cancer and prostate cancer.

You can also protect yourself from heart diseases and degenerative nerve diseases with the help of grapes. Red and purple grapes are rich in nutrients and other plant compounds that can decrease inflammation and lower your risk of disease.

Chapter 6
Low-Cholesterol Recipes

You can manage your blood cholesterol levels by eating food that is low in cholesterol. In this chapter, we will learn different low-cholesterol recipes that could help improve your cholesterol levels by reducing the excess saturated fat and trans-fat.

We should avoid red meat as it can increase the cholesterol level in the blood. We should eat more fish. Vegetables are also a rich source of minerals and vitamins and play a vital role in lowering cholesterol levels.

Do not use solid fats in your recipes; instead, you should use liquid vegetable oils.

Below are some of the low cholesterol recipes which will help lower your cholesterol levels.

1.   **Slow Cooker Picadillo:**

Picadillo is a traditional dish in many Latin-American countries, and it is usually made with ground beef. It also has plenty of spices, including cumin, cinnamon, chili powder, and oregano.

2.   **Sweet Potato Fritters with Smoky Pinto Beans:**

It is a delicious dish and has a crispy crust. The red beans are also delicious and flavored with smoked paprika. In this dish, chili powder is also used as a spice instead of the paprika. It is a high fiber vegetarian dish that is low in cholesterol.

3.   **Chicken and White Bean Salad:**

Chicken and white bean salad is also a very nutritious dish that is low in cholesterol. It is a gluten-free, high fiber dish with many health immunity properties.

4.   **Chicken with Cannellini Beans and Tomato Sauce:**

    Ingredients:

- 1 small red onion chopped
- Olive oil
- 2 garlic cloves
- 1 teaspoon crushed red chili
- 1 chopped tomato
- Cannellini beans
- 2 tablespoons of salted baby capers
- 2 tablespoons chopped continental parsley
- 2 chicken breast fillets
- Steamed green round beans

Preparation Method:

First, heat the saucepan over medium-low heat then spray with olive oil spray to grease. Then put the onion in the pan and stir it occasionally for 4 to 5 minutes. Wait for the onions to become soft. Now, add the garlic, chili, and tomato. Bring to a boil. Add the cannellini beans and capers, and simmer for 5 minutes or until the mixture thickens slightly. Season with pepper. Stir in half the parsley Then cook and stir for one minute until you can smell the aroma.

5. **Penne with Eggplant Caponata:**

It is high in flavor, and it is a tasty dish without any meat.

Ingredients:

- 1 onion chopped
- 2 garlic cloves
- 2 tablespoons olive oil
- 1 large eggplant
- 2 chopped tomatoes
- ½ cup of green olives
- 2 tablespoons caster sugar
- 2 tablespoons chopped flat-leaf parsley
- 400 grams penne rigate
- 1/3 cup drained capers

Preparation Method:

Over medium heat, heat the oil in a pan. Add the onion and garlic in the oil and gently cook it. Stir it for 5 minutes until it becomes a red, light golden color. Now, increase the heat and add eggplant. Then, cook and stir for 2 to 3 minutes until it becomes a golden color. Now, add the tomato, sugar, salt, and pepper.

For 15 minutes, cook over low flame after it is brought to a boil. Then, the eggplant is cooked. The sauce should also thicken at the end. Now, stir in the parsley, olives, and capers.

6.   Lime Spiced Chicken with Pearl Barley and Corn Salad:

Ingredients:

- 60 ml Fresh lime juice
- 2 teaspoons Paprika
- 1 crossed Garlic clove
- 2x200 gram single chicken breast fillets
- 1 cup pearl barley
- Olive oil spray
- 1 ½ cups Sweet corn kernels
- Red capsicum (small and finely chopped)
- 4 shallots (Thin slices)
- ½ cup fresh continental parsley leaves

Preparation Method:

First, mix the lime juice and garlic in a jug. Now, place the chicken in any ceramic dish. Add the remaining lime juice mixture to the chicken and turn to coat. Now place the ceramic dish in the fridge, after covering with plastic wrap, for 20 minutes to marinate. Cook the barley in a saucepan of boiling water until it is tender, then drain all the water. Now, wash it with cold water. Then, heat the pan, spray it with olive oil. Then add the corn and stir it for 2 minutes. Now, add the shallots and capsicum.

Wait for 1 minute. You will see the corn has changed to a light golden color. Add the remaining lime juice into the mixture of corn and parsley. Now, put the marinated chicken in a pan and cook it for 4 minutes. Also, spray it with olive oil spray. Now, slice the chicken thinly. Top the chicken over the barley mixture. It is a very fantastic dish with high-fiber, low-fat, low-sodium, and low-sugar.

7.   Healthy Gumbo:

Gumbo is a very delicious dish and good for your heart. Ingredients in gumbo are fibrous gums and patterns. It is such a fantastic dish that can help lower cholesterol and protect against stomach ulcers.

Ingredients:

- 2 tablespoons canola oil
- 1 medium onion chopped
- 1 medium red paper
- 1 medium green pepper
- 250 grams of okra, cut into 1 cm chunks
- 2 cloves garlic
- 450 mL crushed tomatoes
- 500 mL low-sodium chicken stock
- 500 grams crabmeat
- 1 mL tabasco

Preparation Method:

First, heat oil in a large saucepan over medium-high heat. Now, you can add onion, okra, pepper, and ham. Now, wait for the okra to become soft until it is no longer sticky. Then, wait for 10 minutes. Now you can add garlic and sauce and wait for 1 minute. Add tomatoes and chicken stock mixture. Now, cook it for 20 minutes uncovered. Steam in crab, add tomato, salt, and pepper. Serve it with rice.

Chapter 7

Recipes for Low-Carb and Low-Salt Diets

We should eat low-carbohydrate, and low-salt foods as these are good for health. As we all know, if we consume high-sodium food, there is a risk of blood pressure problems. Our body requires sodium to maintain the balance between body fluids. However, we should consume less salt in our daily life. Similarly, low carb diets limit carbohydrates such as grains, starchy vegetables, and fruit, and contain foods high in protein and fat. There are many essential nutrients present in low-carb diets, including broccoli, asparagus, carrots, cabbage, spinach, mushrooms and much more. Low-carb diets may help prevent or improve serious health conditions, such as metabolic syndrome, diabetes, high blood pressure, and cardiovascular disease. If you follow a low-carbohydrate diet that is higher in fat and possibly higher in protein, it is important to choose food with healthy unsaturated fats and healthy proteins.

1.   **Low-Carb, Low-Sodium Taco Salad:**

Ingredients:

- 1 head of iceberg lettuce, chopped
- 3 tomatoes
- 1 pound of ground beef
- One bunch of scallions, chopped
- One package low-sodium taco seasoning
- 1 cup sharp cheddar cheese
- Optional toppings:
  - ½ cup low sodium black beans
  - ½ cup low sodium corn

Preparation Method:

First, cook the ground beef until it gets brown and drain the fat. Now add 3/4 cup of water and the seasoning spice packet. Wait for the meat to become thickened (until it simmers up).

When the ground beef is getting brown, at the same time, cut all the tomatoes and salad. Also, chop the scallions and cook all the ingredients. When this is ready, then top the salad with cheese and dressing. You can also add beans and corn, but they are optional.

2. **One Skillet Creamy Tuscan Chicken:**

Ingredients:

- 1 ½ cups baby spinach
- ½ cup dried tomatoes
- 2 tablespoons olive oil
- 1 ½ pounds of skinless and boneless chicken breast in slices
- 1 cup cream
- ½ cup low-sodium chicken broth
- 1 teaspoon garlic powder
- 1 teaspoon Italian seasoning
- ½ cup Parmesan cheese
- Chopped fresh parsley

Preparation Method:

First, we will cook the chicken in a large pan over medium heat. Now, we will brown it for about five minutes until it gets a beautiful brown color. Add heavy cream after removing the chicken breast from the pan. Also, add chicken broth, garlic powder, Italian seasoning, and parmesan cheese. Now, mix all the ingredients and simmer for a few minutes.

Now, add sun-dried tomatoes and fresh spinach in the thick cream sauce. Cook the ingredients for about 1 to 2 minutes until the spinach reduces its volume. Put the chicken back in the pan and coat it with the sauce. Now, your delicious Tuscan chicken is ready.

3. **Keto Chaffle Tacos Recipe:**

Ingredients:

- 1 egg
- ½ cup cheddar cheese or mozzarella cheese
- ¼ teaspoon Italian seasoning

Taco Meat Seasoning for Ground Beef:

- 1 teaspoon ground cumin
- 1 teaspoon chili powder
- ½ teaspoon of cocoa powder
- ½ teaspoon garlic powder
- ¼ teaspoon salt
- ½ teaspoon smoked paprika
- ¼ teaspoon onion powder

Preparation Method:

First, we must cook the ground turkey or ground beef. After that add all the taco meat seasonings. You can also add the cocoa powder as it enhances the flavors of all the other seasonings. You can start making the keto chaffles while making Taco meat. Now, preheat the waffle maker and whip the egg in a small bowl.

Then, add the shredded cheese and seasoning. In the mini waffle maker, you can place half the chaffle mixture into it. Now, cook for about 3 to 4 min. Prepare the second half of the mix to make chaffles. Now, you can add the taco meat. Now, repeat and cook the second half of the mixture.

Now, warm taco meat in the taco chaffle. You can also top it with tomatoes, cheese and lettuce. You can also set the tacos standing up so that they hold together. The green sauce on the top of the taco chaffles gives a fantastic look and taste.

Chapter 8
Managing Lifestyle Changes

A lifestyle change will take time and require support. You will have a better life when you make specific positive changes in your life. Nutrition and exercise play a vital role in making favorable changes in your life. In addition to diet and exercise, there are many psychological factors like depression, isolation, loneliness, and anger on which your life depends a lot. Our social health and emotional health are also connected with the reduced risk of disease and premature death. You should have the support and love of your friends and family.

1.   Adopting a Healthy Lifestyle:

We should adopt a healthy lifestyle to bring positive changes in our life. Healthy lifestyle changes are:

- Doing exercise regularly
- Eating healthy food
- Low levels of caffeine and sugar
- Taking a break
- Getting enough sleep
- Asking for help
- Deep breathing
- Reframing problems

2.   How You Can Avoid Stress to Make a Healthy Lifestyle Change:

You need to slow down, let go of worries, avoid people who stress you out. Laugh it up, snooze more, get connected, get organized. Be active, practice giving back, give up the bad habits and focus on things you can change. Manage your time correctly, and you should avoid the last-minute stress. Avoiding cigarettes and exercising regularly is crucial.

3.   Increase Physical Activity:

As we all know, physical activity is significant and will bring remarkable change to our life, and it plays a vital role in removing stress. It improves the health of the person. Physical activity also helps your body to regulate all the hormones. So, the level of hormones is enhanced with the help of physical activity. You should do moderate physical activity for at least 30 minutes a day. If you want to increase your physical activity, brisk walking is also a good option.

4.   Be Willing to Adapt Changes:

"Change is the law of life. And those who look only to the past or the present are certain to miss the future" – John F Kennedy. As this statement reflects, you should adapt to the changes in your life. You need to be prepared for change so that you have control over how you react to the change you are facing in your life. Start by changing your mindset. Once you start to take control of the power of choice, it will enable you to activate positive change in your life. Know what is important in your life and gives you purpose, then set direction on how you want to live your life. Let go of your regrets and move forward in life. Live a balanced, healthy and active life.

5.   You Should Always Have Positive Thinking:

If you are in a problematic situation, then you should look for the brighter side. Positive thinking always plays a significant role in changing your lifestyle. Always go for challenges, as these are the best way for personal growth. You can also learn from your previous experiences. So, do not feel stress in the worst situations. You should find ways to make the situation positive.

6.   Always Do Things Which Are Fun for You:

There should be a time in a busy routine in which you should relax and take a break from all responsibilities. You should always have a sense of humor and connect with other people positively. You can go for a walk with your buddy or soulmate. You can go for lunch with the kids. You can listen to music which relaxes you.

7.   Managing Lifestyle Changes for Heart Attack Prevention:

You should make some changes in your life to prevent yourself from having a heart attack.

- Participate in physical activity
- Choose good nutrition
- Do not smoke
- You should avoid the foods which are high in cholesterol

- Avoid fatty foods
- You should maintain a healthy weight
- Do not put yourself in a stressful condition
- Limit alcohol

## 8.	Managing Lifestyle Changes for Diabetic Patients:

The people who are suffering from diabetes should have some awareness about how to manage diabetes.

- To control the blood sugar levels, always eat healthy things that play a critical role in controlling blood glucose levels.
- Count your carbohydrates and portion size meals
- You should coordinate your meals and medications
- Avoid the juices and drinks which are high in sugar
- Make every meal well-balanced.
- Do physical exercise but make sure that your doctor is aware of your exercise plan.
- Keep an exercise schedule.
- You should check your blood sugar level regularly. Always stay hydrated and be prepared for situations where your blood sugar level drops too low.

Conclusion

With the help of lifestyle changes, you can spend more of your time doing things that you want to do. Adopt good habits starting with changing your diets to have healthy food in your daily routine. Do any type of physical activity for a minimum of 30 minutes daily to stay healthy as regular physical activity is good for your health. If you do have a setback, do not give up but persevere. Setbacks happen to everyone. Regroup and focus on meeting your goals again as soon as you can.

Lastly, I wish you good health, and I hope you have a balanced and positive lifestyle. Thank you for reading this eBook.

-- Katherine Young